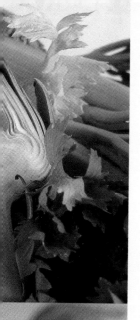

# introduction

Eating foods that promote good health makes sense, and is surprisingly simple. If you already eat a well-balanced diet, you'll have a head start. Making sensible choices, like eating plenty of starchy carbohydrates, only moderate amounts of protein foods and lots of fruit and vegetables will come naturally. You will like your meat lean and your fish oily – most of the time – and will limit the amount of salt, sugar and fat you consume. You'll eat about three servings of low-fat dairy produce daily, and drink plenty of water. You'll enjoy cooking, and trying new foods, especially if they offer all-round benefits to your health, or have the potential to ease distressing symptoms of ill health.

That's what this book is about: tapping into current scientific knowledge about healing foods and taking advantage of new discoveries. There's never been a more exciting time in the world of nutrition, and the benefits are there for all of us.

# eating for good health

**What we eat has a profound effect on our health and well-being. In a world that is becoming increasingly polluted, and where individuals are subject to high levels of stress, it is easy for our bodies to become out of kilter.**

There is ample evidence of a link between poor diet and serious medical conditions like coronary heart disease, cancer and strokes, but it is not just these major health problems that we should be concerned about. A health condition does not have to be life threatening to have a huge impact on the way we feel.

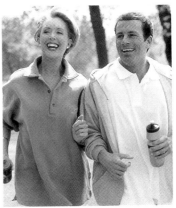

▲ INCORPORATING EXERCISE INTO YOUR DAILY ROUTINE WILL HELP YOU LOOK AND FEEL YOUNGER AND FITTER.

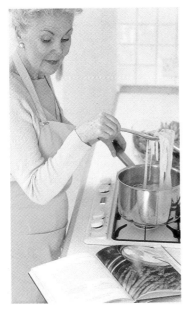

Whatever ails us, whether it is the occasional headache or sore throat, an ongoing condition like diabetes or a digestive problem that causes embarrassment and distress, specific foods can have a positive impact when eaten as part of a sensible, well-balanced diet.

◀ TRYING OUT NEW, HEALTHY RECIPES IS BOTH REWARDING AND ENJOYABLE.

▶ A LOW-FAT MEDITERRANEAN DIET CONSISTING OF FISH, FRESH VEGETABLES AND FRUIT, OLIVE OIL AND A SMALL AMOUNT OF RED WINE PROMOTES GOOD CIRCULATION.

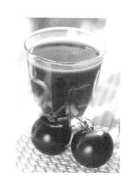

# healing with
# food

A concise guide to using
the therapeutic properties
of food to stay healthy and
fight infection

## JENNI FLEETWOOD

HERMES
HOUSE

The edition published by Hermes House

© Anness Publishing Limited 2002 updated 2003..

Hermes House is an imprint of Anness Publishing Limited,
Hermes House, 88–89 Blackfriars Road, London SE1 8HA

Publisher: Joanna Lorenz
Production Controller: Joanna King

Publisher's Note:
The Reader should not regard the recommendations, ideas and techniques
expressed and described in this book as substitutes for the advice of a
qualified medical practitioner or other qualified professional.
Any use to which the recommendations, ideas and techniques
are put is at the reader's sole discretion and risk.

Printed in Hong Kong/China

3 5 7 9 10 8 6 4

# contents

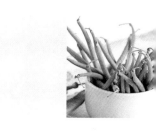

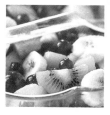

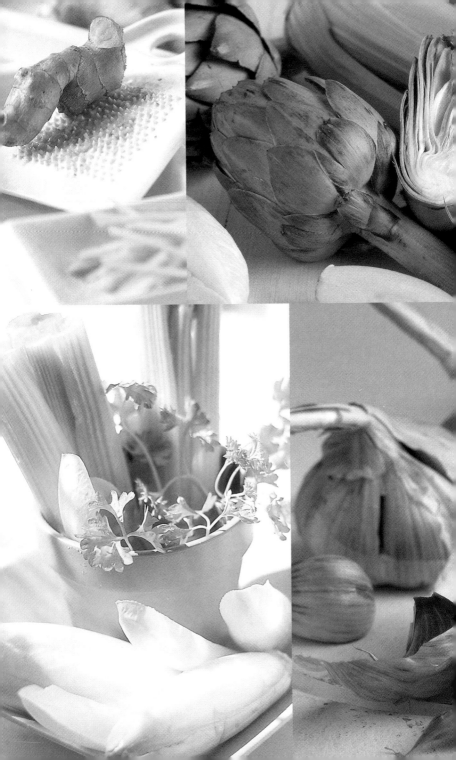

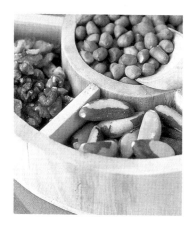

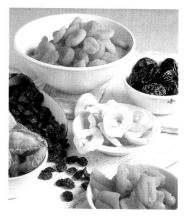

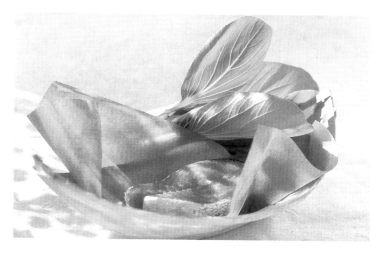

▲ LEFT AND RIGHT: CHOOSE HEALTHY SNACKS THAT NURTURE YOUR BODY, INSTEAD OF REACHING FOR SNACKS WITH EMPTY CALORIES.

Making relatively small changes to our diet, such as eating fruit for a mid-morning snack, can improve matters considerably.

It is important to seek professional advice from a doctor, nutritionist, dietician or state-registered medical specialist before making major changes to your diet, particularly if you are taking any kind of medication.

# superfoods

Some foods are such a rich source of concentrated nutrients that they have earned themselves the title "superfoods". Some, such as tofu, are old favourites; others, such as quinoa, have only recently received widespread acclaim.

To understand why these foods are so special, it is useful to look at recent scientific research. One of the most exciting discoveries has been the presence in plants of thousands of different chemical compounds. Each of these compounds – known collectively as phytochemicals – has its own function, and it is believed that some of them may play a crucial role in preventing diseases like cancer, heart disease, arthritis and hypertension. To get the best benefit from phytochemicals, eat at least five different types of fruit and vegetables daily, plus wholegrains, pulses, nuts and seeds.

▼ BUY VEGETABLES IN SMALL QUANTITIES AND EAT THEM AT THEIR FRESHEST.

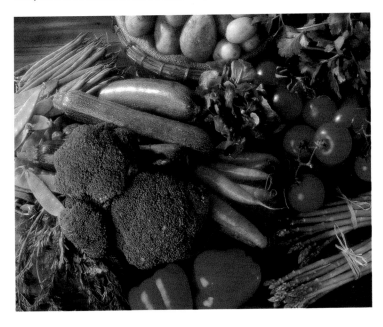

A number of phyto-chemicals also have antioxidant proper-ties. Antioxidants are vital for limiting damage to body cells by unstable molecules known as free radicals. The main antioxidant nutri-ents are vitamins A, C and E, and the minerals zinc and selenium.

When we chew, our bodies produce enzymes. These are protein molecules and are responsible for every aspect of metabolism or the energy we produce. Producing plenty of enzymes improves digestion, detox-ification and immunity, and helps to slow down the ageing process.

◀ QUINOA (LEFT) IS A COMPLETE PROTEIN AND HAS A MILD, SLIGHTLY BITTER TASTE AND FIRM TEXTURE. COOK IT IN THE SAME WAY AS RICE. MILLET (BELOW) IS A HIGHLY NUTRITIOUS GLUTEN-FREE GRAIN.

Many of the superfoods highlighted in the pages that follow are excellent sources of enzymes and phytochemicals. Others are included because they contribute valuable minerals, vitamins or omega-3 fatty acids, which are important allies in reducing the risk of heart disease.

▼ STRAWBERRIES ARE RICH IN B COMPLEX VITAMINS AND VITAMIN C. THEY CONTAIN SIGNIFICANT AMOUNTS OF POTASSIUM, AND HAVE GOOD SKIN-CLEANSING PROPERTIES.

## GOOD SOURCES OF ANTIOXIDANTS
- Sweet potatoes
- Carrots
- Watercress
- Broccoli
- Peas
- Citrus fruit
- Watermelon
- Strawberries
- Nuts and Seeds

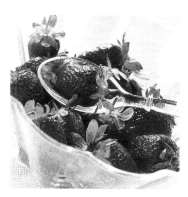

# fruit

**What easier way to help yourself to good health than to eat plenty of fruit? There are so many different varieties, with glowing colours and delectable flavours, that eating the recommended portions daily is pure pleasure.**

For maximum nutrition, eat fruit that is ripe and freshly picked, and choose lots of different varieties, as each offers many different benefits.

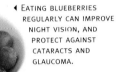

◀ EATING BLUEBERRIES REGULARLY CAN IMPROVE NIGHT VISION, AND PROTECT AGAINST CATARACTS AND GLAUCOMA.

Fruit provides soluble fibre in the form of pectin, which aids digestion and helps to cleanse the liver. All fruits contain generous quantities of antioxidant vitamins C and E, phytochemicals and beta-carotene, which the body converts to vitamin A. They help to prevent the furring up of the arteries that leads to atherosclerosis and, in addition, support the

▼ SUMMER PRODUCES AN ABUNDANT CROP OF DELICIOUS SOFT FRUITS.

▼ FRUIT IS THE ULTIMATE CONVENIENCE FOOD, AND AN EXCELLENT SOURCE OF FIBRE.

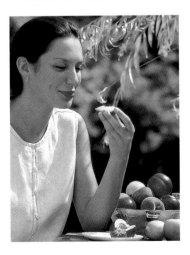

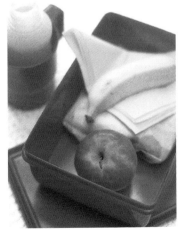

▶ BLACKCURRANTS ARE USUALLY SERVED COOKED AND HAVE A TART FLAVOUR.

body's defence system. The antioxidants in fruit may also ease the discomfort of arthritis sufferers by mopping up free radicals and helping to promote the growth of new cartilage. Mangoes, apricots, apples and bananas are particularly useful in this regard.

**Apples** contain the flavonoid quercetin, which may reduce the risk of heart attacks and strokes.

**Bananas** are a good source of fibre, vitamins and minerals, especially potassium, which is important for nerve, cell and muscle function, and can help to relieve high blood pressure. Bananas have a high starch content so provide sustained energy. They are a source of tryptophan, an amino acid that lifts the spirits and aids sleep. Ripe bananas strengthen the stomach lining against acid and ulcers.

**Blackcurrants** are high in antioxidants, vitamins C and E, and carotenes. They contain fibre, and the minerals calcium, iron and

▼ FRESH FRUIT SALAD IS A HEALTHY AND NUTRITIOUS DESSERT.

## HOW MUCH IS A PORTION?

Nutritionists recommend eating five portions of fruit and vegetables a day, but what is a portion?

• One medium apple, banana or orange
• A wine glass of any fresh fruit juice
• One large slice of any type of melon or pineapple
• Two plums or kiwi fruit
• About 115g/4oz/1 cup berries

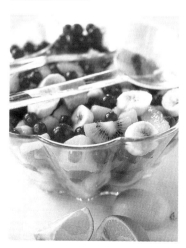

▶ GOOSEBERRIES ARE A RICH SOURCE OF VITAMIN C.

magnesium. Blackcurrants are useful for treating stomach upsets.

**Citrus fruits, melons and kiwi fruit** are rich in vitamin C, offering relief to asthmatics and people suffering from a wide range of respiratory problems. The membranes of citrus fruit contain pectin, which helps to reduce cholesterol, and also bioflavonoids, which have powerful antioxidant properties.

**Figs** have laxative qualities and are a good source of calcium.

**Gooseberries** are rich in vitamin C and also contain betacarotene, potassium and fibre.

**Mangoes and apricots** contain betacarotene, which may help to prevent inflammation of the lungs and airways. Mangoes are reputed to cleanse the blood, while apricots are a valuable source of vitamin A.

**Papaya** or pawpaw contains an enzyme called papain, which aids digestion. This fruit contains vitamin C, promoting healthy skin, hair and nails.

**Raspberries** are a rich source of vitamin C. Eat them to alleviate menstrual cramps. They cleanse the body and remove harmful toxins.

**Strawberries** cleanse the skin. They are rich in B complex vitamins and vitamin C.

**Tomatoes** ripened on the vine have higher levels of vitamin C than those picked when green. They contain vitamin E, betacarotene, magnesium, calcium and phosphorus. They aid digestion, reduce blood pressure and lower the risk of developing asthma. Tomatoes contain lycopene, which is believed to prevent some forms of cancer.

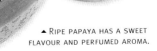

▲ RIPE PAPAYA HAS A SWEET FLAVOUR AND PERFUMED AROMA.

## RECIPE SUGGESTION

Baked Apples

For a nutritious dessert, try these tasty baked apples stuffed with dried fruit and nuts.

*Ingredients*

*4 cooking apples*

*115g/4oz/²⁄₃ cup mixed dried fruit and nuts*

*20ml/4 tsp soft dark brown sugar*

*butter*

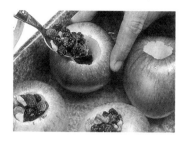

**1** Preheat the oven to 180°C/350°F/Gas 4. Remove the core from the apples, score them round their middles, then place them in a baking dish.

**2** Mix the fruit, nuts and sugar together and fill the centre of each apple. Pour a little water around the apples and top each with a knob (pat) of butter.

**3** Bake for 40–60 minutes, until soft and golden. Serve hot, with low-fat yogurt. Serves 4.

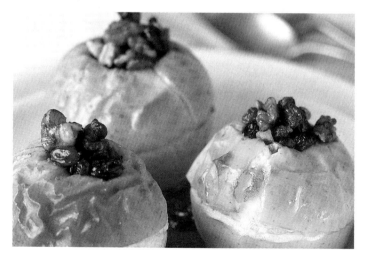

# vegetables

**One of the easiest ways of boosting your intake of fibre, vitamins and minerals is to eat plenty of vegetables. Buy organic produce where possible, and make sure it is fresh by purchasing produce from a store with a fast turnover.**

Box schemes, run by independent suppliers or co-operatives, are an excellent idea. You state how much you want to spend and how often you would like a delivery, and boxes of beautiful produce arrive on your doorstep regularly. You may be able to specify what they contain, but it can be more fun to have a little of whatever is being harvested. That way you get to try some unfamiliar vegetables.

Like fruit, all vegetables contain phytochemicals, the plant compounds that stimulate the body's enzyme defences against carcinogens (the substances that cause cancer). The best sources are broccoli, cabbages, kohlrabi, radishes, cauliflower, Brussels sprouts, watercress, turnips, kale, pak choi (bok choy), mustard greens, spring

▼ CRUCIFEROUS VEGETABLES ARE PACKED WITH PHYTOCHEMICALS.

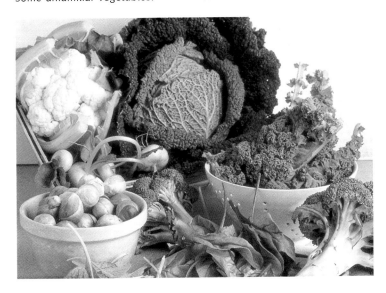

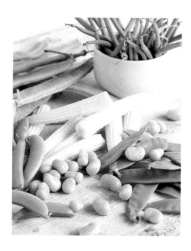

▲ Beans, peas and corn can be enjoyed all year round, fresh or frozen.

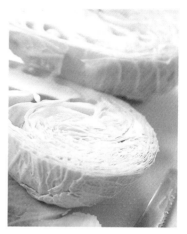

▲ Cabbage is best eaten raw. It is a valuable source of vitamins C and E.

greens (collards), chard and swede (rutabaga). Vegetables are also a good source of antioxidants.

**Artichokes** are good liver cleansers. A source of vitamins A and C, fibre, iron, calcium and potassium, they are used in natural medicine to treat high blood pressure.

**Asparagus** has anti-inflammatory properties and helps to soothe painful joints.

**Beetroot (beet)**, when eaten raw, helps to cleanse the liver and is good for detoxifying the skin.

**Cabbage** has antiviral and antibacterial qualities and is particularly useful raw or juiced. It is thought to speed up the metabolism of oestrogen in women and may protect against breast cancer or cancer of the womb.

**Carrots and sweet potatoes** are rich in betacarotene, which may help to prevent inflammation of the lungs and airways, and may also ease painful conditions of the joints, such as arthritis.

**Chillies** are very high in vitamin C. They can help to thin mucus and relieve congested airways, and also stimulate the circulation.

**Fennel** aids digestion, is a diuretic and has a calming and toning effect on the stomach.

**Garlic** has been found to lower blood cholesterol levels, reduce

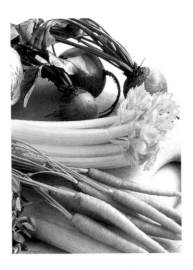

▲ CARROTS AND BEETROOT (BEET) HELP THE LIVER TO DETOXIFY THE BODY.

possibly prevent asthma attacks. Onions also contain quercetin, an anti-inflammatory that can ease painful joints.

**Peas and beans** are a good source of protein and fibre. They also contain vitamin C, iron, thiamine, folate, phosphorous and potassium.

**Peppers** contain plenty of vitamin C, as well as betacarotene, some B complex vitamins, calcium, phosphorous and iron.

**Salad leaves** are largely composed of water, but are worth eating for

blood pressure and help to prevent the formation of blood clots. An antiviral and antibacterial allium, garlic strengthens the immune system. It is a nasal decongestant. It is best eaten raw, but cooking does not radically decrease its decongestant properties.

**Green vegetables** that are rich in folic acid may help to lower the risk of heart disease by reducing levels of the amino acid, homocysteine. (High levels are linked to increased risk of coronary heart disease.)

**Onions** have long been considered a folk cure for respiratory problems. They help clear the airways and

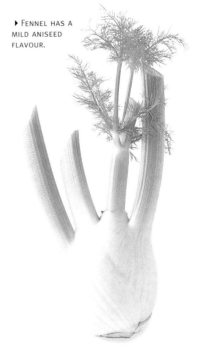

▸ FENNEL HAS A MILD ANISEED FLAVOUR.

## POP A PEA

Peas are unusual in that the frozen ones are often more nutritious than fresh store-bought ones, thanks to the super-efficient harvesting methods that mean they are frozen on the day they are picked.

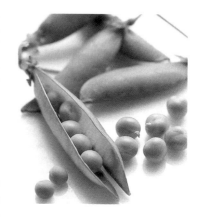

the vitamins and minerals they contribute to the diet. Choose the outer, darker leaves of lettuces, as they are more nutritious than the pale leaves in the centre.

**Spinach** is a rich source of cancer-fighting antioxidants, fibre and vitamins C and B6. It also contains calcium, potassium, folate, thiamine, zinc and four times more betacarotene than broccoli.

▲ PEAS PICKED AND EATEN FRESH FROM THE POD HAVE A DELICIOUS SWEET TASTE.

▼ ASPARAGUS HAS MILD DIURETIC AND LAXATIVE PROPERTIES.

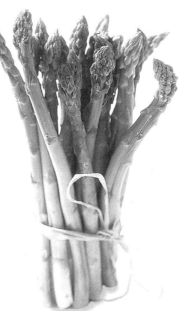

▼ GARLIC IMPARTS A STRONGER FLAVOUR INTO COOKING WHEN USED CRUSHED.

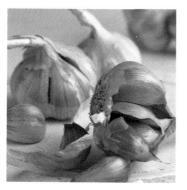

# sprouted grains, seeds & pulses

Sprouted seeds are powerhouses of nutrition. Once the seed, pulse or grain germinates, the nutritional value rockets – by as much as 30 per cent in the case of B vitamins, and 60 per cent for vitamin C.

Sprouts supply plenty of protein, vitamin E, potassium and phosphorus. You can buy sprouts from supermarkets, but they'll be fresher – and cost less – if you grow them. Children love watching them germinate, they taste good in fresh and cooked dishes, and they are very easy to digest.

Many seeds, pulses (legumes) and grains can be sprouted successfully. Here are some of the best.

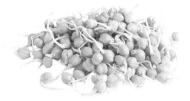

▲ CHICKPEA SPROUTS.

**Chickpea sprouts** are deliciously nutty, but take longer to sprout than small beans. They must be rinsed four times a day.

▼ LENTIL SPROUTS.

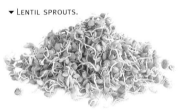

**Lentil sprouts** are slightly spicy and peppery. Use whole (not split) red,

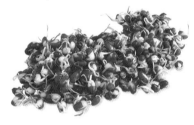

▲ ADUKI BEANSPROUTS.

**Aduki beansprouts** are said to be good for cleansing the system. These fine, feathery sprouts have a sweet, nutty flavour.
**Alfalfa sprouts** are wispy little sprouts with a nutty, mild flavour. They are best eaten raw.

▼ ALFALFA SPROUTS.

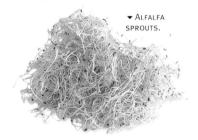

green and brown lentils. They are best eaten when young.

▼ Mung beansprouts.

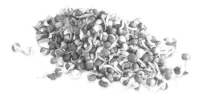

**Mung beansprouts** are large, with a delicate flavour and crunchy texture. They are great in salads.

▼ Wheat berry sprouts.

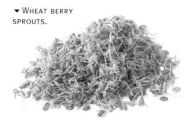

**Wheat berry sprouts** are sweet and crunchy. They taste great in breads.

## Storing Sprouts

Use sprouts as soon as possible after growing or buying. If you must store them, put them in a plastic bag or sealed tub in the refrigerator. They will keep for 2–3 days. Wash and drain bought sprouts before using them.

## SPROUTING

There's nothing simpler than sprouting seeds. It's the fastest way to grow your own organic produce. Most seeds are ready to eat in 3–4 days.

**1** Rinse 45ml/3 tbsp seeds, pulses (legumes) or grains, drain and place in a clean jar. Fill with lukewarm water, cover with muslin and fasten securely. Leave in a warm place overnight.

**2** Pour off the water, leaving the muslin in place. Refill with water, shake gently, then drain as before. Leave the jar in a warm place, away from direct sunlight.

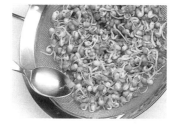

**3** Rinse and drain three times a day until they have grown to the desired size. Remove from the jar, rinse, drain and discard any that haven't germinated.

# sea vegetables

For centuries, Asian cooks have known about the health benefits of sea vegetables such as arame, laver and kombu, but the Western world is just waking up to the potential of including these valuable superfoods in the diet.

Sea vegetables are an excellent source of betacarotene and contain some of the B complex vitamins. They are rich in minerals. Calcium, magnesium, potassium, phosphorus and iron are all present, and are credited with boosting the immune system, reducing stress and helping the metabolism to function efficiently. Eating sea vegetables regularly can improve the hair and skin, and the iodine they contribute improves thyroid function and prevents goitre.

Sea vegetables can be used in many different ways. Try toasting them and crumbling them into stir-fries or salads, or add them to soups and casseroles.

**Arame** is sold as thin, wiry strips. It is mild and slightly sweet.

**Dulse** is a purple-red sea vegetable which is chewy and tastes spicy. It is rich in potassium, iodine, phosphorous, iron and manganese.

◄ ARAME.

**Kombu** is an essential ingredient in the Japanese stock, dashi. It has a strong flavour and is a rich source of iodine.

**Laver** is a rich source of minerals and vitamins. Cans of laver purée are available from health food stores. Spread it on hot toast.

**Nori** is a delicately flavoured seaweed that is processed into thin sheets, to be used as wraps. Toast it under a grill (broiler) before use.

**Wakame** is a versatile sea vegetable, rich in calcium and vitamins B and C. It can also be toasted and crumbled over food.

▼ DULSE.

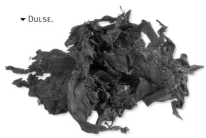

## RECIPE SUGGESTION

SIMPLE SALMON SUSHI

Sushi is a healthy snack. The rice contributes complex carbohydrate, the fish is a good source of protein and omega-3 fatty acids, and the nori wrapper is a source of iodine.

*INGREDIENTS*

*25ml/1½ tbsp granulated sugar*
*5ml/1 tsp sea salt*
*30ml/2 tbsp Japanese rice vinegar*
*250g/9oz/1¼ cups sushi rice*
*3 sheets yaki nori (toasted nori)*
*175g/6oz very fresh salmon fillet, cut into fingers*

**1** Mix the sugar and salt in a bowl. Add the vinegar and stir until dissolved.

**2** Cook the rice according to the instructions on the packet. Drain, add the vinegar mixture and stir well, fanning the rice constantly. Cover with a damp cloth. Cool.

**3** Cut the yaki nori in half lengthways and place a half-sheet, shiny side down, on a bamboo mat.

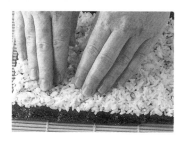

**4** Spread with a layer of vinegared rice, leaving a 1cm/½in clear edge at top and bottom. Arrange fingers of salmon across the centre.

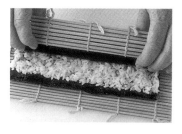

**5** Roll up the yaki nori into a cigar. Wrap in clear film and chill.

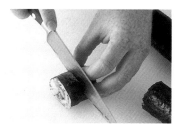

**6** Cut into 24 slices.

# cereal grains

**The seeds of cereal grasses, grains are packed with concentrated goodness and are an important source of complex carbohydrates, protein, vitamins and minerals. Grains are inexpensive and versatile.**

Wheat, rice, oats and barley have always been an important part of the diet, but it is some of the less well-known grains that are currently causing excitement. Two of these are quinoa and millet. Both have been cultivated for centuries, but it is only comparatively recently that the full extent of their nutritional value has been realized.

**Millet** is highly nutritious. Low in fat, it is easily digested. The grains are a good source of iron, zinc, calcium, manganese and B vitamins.

**Oats** have been found to lower blood pressure. They provide insoluble fibre, which can reduce blood cholesterol levels when part of a low-fat diet. Oats are a source of vitamin E, an anti-inflammatory.

**Quinoa** is the only grain that is a complete protein, possessing all eight essential amino acids. Low in saturated fats and high in fibre, it is an excellent source of calcium, potassium, zinc, iron, magnesium and B vitamins. It is cooked like rice, but the grains swell to four times their original size. As the grain cooks, the germ that surrounds it forms a spiral that resembles a bean sprout. This stays firm and crunchy, providing a tasty contrast to the soft, creamy grain. Use quinoa in pilaffs, bakes, stuffings and as a breakfast cereal. It is also available in flakes and as flour.

◀ CLOCKWISE FROM TOP: ROLLED OATS, OATMEAL, WHOLE OATS AND OATBRAN.

**Wheat** is a nutritious grain, but not everyone can tolerate it. It is best eaten unprocessed, as wholewheat. It is a very good source of dietary fibre, most of which is in the bran. It also contains B vitamins, vitamin E, iron, selenium and zinc. Wholegrains are a source of phytoestrogens, which may also help to protect against breast cancer.

**Rice** is a good source of fibre, vitamins and minerals. Eat brown rice where possible, as it retains the husk, bran and germ in which most of the nutrients reside.

## RECIPE SUGGESTION

TABBOULEH

A quick and easy way to boost your dietary fibre intake.

*INGREDIENTS*

*175g/6oz/1 cup bulgur wheat*
*30ml/2 tbsp each chopped fresh*
  *mint and parsley*
*6 spring onions (scallions), sliced*
*½ cucumber, diced*
*60ml/4 tbsp extra virgin olive oil*
*juice of 1 large lemon*
*salt and ground black pepper*

**1** Place the bulgur wheat in a bowl. Pour on boiling water to cover. Leave to stand for 30 minutes, so that the grains swell.

**2** Drain well, removing as much water as possible. Tip the wheat into a bowl.

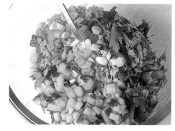

**3** Add all the remaining ingredients and toss well. Chill for 30 minutes to allow the flavours to mingle. Serve as a salad, or as a filling for warm wheat tortillas, with guacamole. Serves 4–6.

# pulses

**Low in fat and high in complex carbohydrates, vitamins and minerals, pulses are economical, easy to cook and good to eat. They are a valuable source of protein and good for diabetics, as they help to control sugar levels.**

LENTILS AND DRIED PEAS

There are several varieties. All these pulses (legumes) are low in fat and rich in protein. They are a good source of fibre and are reputed to help lower levels of harmful LDL cholesterol.

▼ YELLOW AND GREEN SPLIT PEAS.

DRIED BEANS

These are packed with protein, soluble and insoluble fibre, iron, potassium, manganese, magnesium, folate and most B vitamins. Soya beans are the superfood here, containing all the amino acids essential for the renewal of cells and tissues. Including dried beans in your diet regularly can lower cholesterol levels, reducing the risk of heart disease and strokes. Beans contain phytoestrogens, which can protect against cancer of the breast, prostate and colon. There are plenty of other varieties too, including aduki beans, black beans, black-eyed beans (peas), borlotti beans, broad (fava) beans, butter (lima) beans, flageolet or cannellini beans, chickpeas, haricot (navy) beans, pinto beans, red kidney beans and ful medames. Canned beans are not as nutritious as dried beans, but contain appreciable amounts of nutrients.

◀ CLOCKWISE FROM LEFT: HARICOT (NAVY) BEANS, KIDNEY BEANS, FLAGEOLET (CANNELLINI) BEANS AND PINTO BEANS.

SPLIT PEA MASH

This purée makes an excellent alternative to mashed potatoes, and is particularly good with winter pies and nut roasts. Serve warm with pitta bread.

*INGREDIENTS*

*225g/8oz/1 cup yellow split peas, soaked overnight*
*1 bay leaf*
*8 sage leaves, roughly chopped*
*15ml/1 tbsp olive oil*
*4 shallots, finely chopped*
*5ml/1 tsp cumin seeds*
*1 large garlic clove, chopped*
*50g/2oz/¼ cup butter, softened*
*salt and ground black pepper*

**1** Drain the split peas, put them in a pan with cold water to cover and bring to the boil. Skim, add the herbs and simmer for 10 minutes.

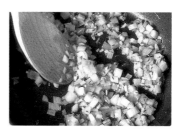

**2** Heat the oil and fry the shallots with the cumin seeds and garlic for 3 minutes. Add to the pan and simmer for 30 minutes more. Drain, reserving the cooking water.

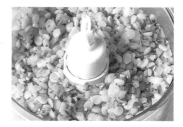

**3** Remove the bay leaf, then process the split peas with the butter and enough of the cooking water to form a coarse purée. Season, serve warm with diced tomatoes and olive oil. Serves 4–6.

# protein foods

**An essential nutrient, protein is converted by the body into amino acids, which are vital for the growth and repair of body cells. The body manufactures some amino acids, but eight cannot be manufactured.**

Eating a good variety of proteins is important because the eight amino acids have to come from our food. The other 12 amino acids can all be synthesised from the food that we eat. Good sources of protein are red meat, poultry, fish, milk, eggs, quinoa, lentils and beans, especially soya beans and their derivatives. Tofu, an excellent source of protein, is a rich source of B vitamins, essential fatty acids,

▼ EAT A VARIETY OF PROTEIN TO ENSURE YOU GET THE MAXIMUM NUTRIENTS.

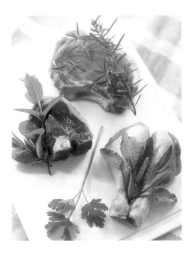

zinc and iron. It contains phyto-estrogens that help to regulate hormone levels, and can lower cholesterol levels if eaten regularly.

Although protein is so important, we do not need to eat vast amounts of it; eating too much protein, especially animal protein, can lead to weight gain and osteoporosis. Far better to balance a moderate amount of animal protein with protein from plant sources, such as tofu, quinoa, rice and pasta. There is also protein in bread and breakfast cereals.

Limit red meat to four 115–175g/ 4–6oz servings a week, and try not to eat more than three eggs. Milk, cheese and yogurt provide protein, calcium and vitamins B12, A and D. Choose low-fat products and consume in moderation.

Eat fish twice a week. Choose oily fish for preference. Herrings, sardines, mackerel, salmon and tuna provide omega-3 fatty acids, which can help to reduce the risk of heart disease.

## RECIPE SUGGESTION

MOROCCAN SPICED MACKEREL
A spicy marinade is the perfect foil for rich, oily fish.

*INGREDIENTS*
*150ml/¼ pint/⅔ cup sunflower oil*
*15ml/1 tbsp paprika*
*5–10ml/1–2 tsp chilli powder*
*10ml/2 tsp ground cumin*
*10ml/2 tsp ground coriander*
*2 garlic cloves, crushed*
*juice of 2 lemons*
*30ml/2 tbsp chopped fresh mint*
*30ml/2 tbsp chopped fresh coriander (cilantro)*
*4 mackerel, cleaned*
*salt and ground black pepper*
*lemon wedges and mint sprigs, to serve*

**1** Whisk the oil, spices, garlic and lemon juice. Add the herbs.

**2** Slash each mackerel in several places, then place in the dish. Turn to coat in the marinade.

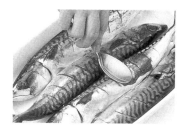

**3** Cover with plastic wrap and chill for 3–5 hours. Grill (broil) for 5–7 minutes on each side. Turn once and baste often. Serve with lemon and mint. Serves 4.

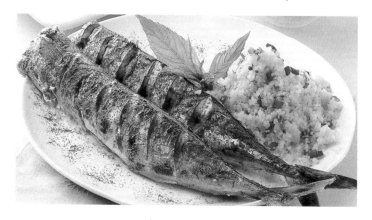

# nuts & seeds

Seeds and nuts make a valuable addition to the diet. Most nuts make delicious snacks, and are tasty sprinkled on salads and desserts. A few almonds, dry-roasted in a frying pan, make a wonderful topping for grilled chicken.

Nuts are an excellent source of B complex vitamins and vitamin E, an antioxidant that has been associated with a lower risk of heart disease, stroke and certain cancers. They are a useful source of protein, but are high in calories, so don't have too many of them.

WALNUTS. ▾

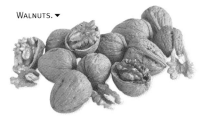

### In a Nutshell

**Brazil nuts** are high in saturated fat, but cholesterol-free. They are a rich source of selenium, which is a mood enhancer.

**Chestnuts** contain very little fat and are a good source of potassium.

**Peanuts** are high in fat, but a good source of potassium. Eat sparingly.

**Pecan nuts** have a very high fat content, so eat only occasionally.

**Walnuts** supply omega-3 fatty acids, which help to keep the heart healthy. Fatty acids thin the blood, which helps to prevent blood clots (DVT) and reduce blood cholesterol levels. They can also reduce inflammation in painful joints. Walnuts are also rich in potassium, magnesium, iron, zinc, copper and selenium.

▾ Unsalted nuts of any kind make a healthy snack for any time of day.

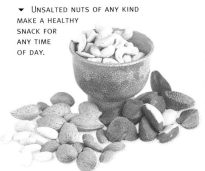

## Caution
• Always inform guests if you've included nuts in a dish, as some people are highly allergic to them.
• Never eat rancid nuts, as they have been linked to a high incidence of free radicals.

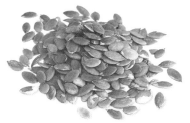

▲ Pumpkin seeds.

## Seed Catalogue

Packed with vitamins and minerals, as well as beneficial oils and protein, seeds make delicious snacks, or can be sprinkled over food to boost the nutritional benefits.

**Linseed** has abundant levels of omega-3 and omega-6 fatty acids, good for strengthening immunity and easing digestive problems.

**Pumpkin seeds** are rich in iron and an excellent source of zinc.

**Sesame seeds** are tiny white or black seeds and are rich in iron.

**Sunflower seeds** are delicious when dry-roasted. They are a good source of vitamin E and B vitamins and boost flagging energy levels.

▼ Linseeds (left) and hemp seeds.

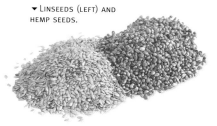

### RECIPE SUGGESTION

Salad and Roasted Seeds
A nutritious light lunch or supper dish.

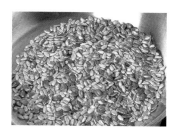

1 Dry-fry 50g/2oz/6 tbsp mixed pumpkin seeds and sunflower seeds in a frying pan, over a high heat, for 3 minutes until golden, tossing frequently to stop them from burning. Set aside to cool slightly.

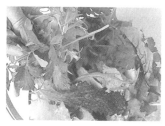

2 Mix about 175g/6oz salad and herb leaves in a bowl. Add the roasted seeds and toss with 30ml/2 tbsp vinaigrette to combine. Serves 4.

# herbs & spices

Herbs and spices are invaluable in the kitchen, not only because they help to make our food taste good without the need for excessive amounts of salt, but also because they are healing foods. Many herbs aid digestion.

**Basil** helps to relieve stomach cramps, nausea and constipation.

**Chillies** are an excellent source of vitamin C and a good source of other antioxidants. The spice stimulates the body and is a powerful decongestant.

**Cinnamon** aids digestion.

**Fennel** calms the digestive system.

**Ginger** is an expectorant that helps to fight coughs and colds. It also soothes stomach cramps. Fresh root ginger is an anti-inflammatory, and may help to ease painful joints.

**Parsley** delivers betacarotene, vitamin B12, ample amounts of vitamin C and a host of minerals, including iron. It aids digestion, can be used as a breath freshener, purifies

◄ ROSEMARY AND SAGE.

the blood and supports the liver and the kidneys.

**Peppermint** is good for digestive problems. A tisane of peppermint and basil can alleviate flatulence.

**Rosemary** tea is effective against cold symptoms, fatigue and headaches.

**Sage** is an antiseptic, antibacterial herb. Sage tea eases indigestion and menopausal problems.

**Turmeric** is an earthy spice that is valued for its antibacterial and anti-fungal properties. Including it in the diet may reduce the risk of certain cancers. It has anti-inflammatory properties, and may ease painful joints.

▼ CHILLIES.

▲ PARSLEY.

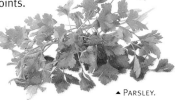

# foods to avoid

**Cut down on foods that are high in saturated fat, including high-fat dairy products, fatty meat and hydrogenated or trans fats found in margarine and processed foods. Drink alcohol in moderation and eat less salt.**

If you have respiratory problems, avoid wine, beer, cider, salt, dairy products, wheat, food additives, yeast and red meat. For a weak or compromised immune system, avoid or eat in moderation, dairy products, caffeine, alcohol and processed foods. To ease digestive problems, avoid bran, spicy foods, alcohol and processed foods.

Arthritis sufferers may benefit from cutting down on or eliminating saturated fat and acidic foods, such as citrus fruits. Caffeine, red meat, sugar, alcohol, aubergines (eggplant), tomatoes and potatoes can exacerbate symptoms, so try eliminating these by degrees.

If you are anxious or stressed, avoid or cut down on stimulants, including nicotine, which can deplete the body of valuable nutrients. Alcohol leads to dehydration, and robs the body of vitamins A and C, B vitamins, magnesium, zinc and essential fatty acids. Tea and coffee inhibit the absorption of iron, magnesium and calcium.

▼ ALCOHOL CAN INHIBIT THE ABSORPTION OF ESSENTIAL VITAMINS AND MINERALS.

▼ CUT DOWN ON THE AMOUNT OF SATURATED FATS THAT YOU EAT.

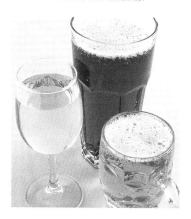

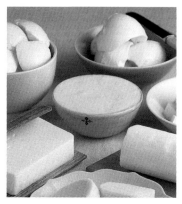

# maximizing nutritional value

**To get the most nutritional value from your food, especially fruit and vegetables, it should be as fresh as possible, and any preparation or cooking should ensure that as many nutrients as possible are retained.**

• If you grow your own fruit and vegetables, or buy from a farm where the produce is picked or pulled as needed, freshness is guaranteed. If not, make sure your supplier has a rapid turnover.

• Transport produce home quickly. Remove any plastic wrapping. Store produce in a cool larder or in the refrigerator crisper.

• Avoid buying fresh produce from a supermarket or store that has installed fluorescent lighting over displays, as this can cause a chemical reaction, depleting nutrients in fruit and vegetables.

• Buy organic produce where possible, and do not peel it unless absolutely necessary, since nutrients are concentrated just below the skin. Instead wash produce thoroughly. Although prepared vegetables are convenient, it is not a good idea to peel or slice

▼ BUY LOOSE PRODUCE WHEN YOU CAN: IT IS EASIER TO CHECK THAN PRE-PACKED FOOD.

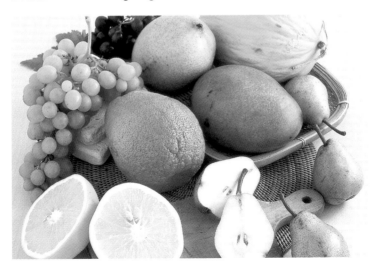

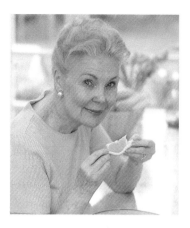

▲ An orange a day supplies an adult with the daily requirement of vitamin C.

produce until you are ready to use it, as the nutritional value diminishes rapidly after preparation.

• Try to eat most of your vegetables and fruit raw. Otherwise, use a steamer in preference to boiling vegetables since soluble vitamins, such as thiamine and vitamin C and B vitamins leach into the water. If you must boil vegetables, use just a little water, and save the water to use in a soup or sauce.

• Buy nuts and seeds in small quantities. Store them in airtight containers in a cool, dark place. Herbs, spices, pulses (legumes), flours and grains should be kept in the same way. Store oils in a cool, dark place to prevent oxidation.

## STORAGE TIPS

**Apples** Store in a cool place, away from direct sunlight.

**Bananas** Store bananas at cool room temperature, away from other fruit.

**Berries** Store in a tub lined with a paper towel, in the refrigerator. Use the same day if possible.

**Celery** Store in the salad drawer of the refrigerator for 1–2 weeks.

**Fennel** Keep for 2–3 days in the salad drawer of the refrigerator.

**Grapes** Store unwashed in the refrigerator for up to 5 days.

**Squash** Can be kept for several weeks in a cool, dry place. When cut, wrap and store in refrigerator.

**Tomatoes** Store at room temperature; chilling spoils the taste and texture.

▼ To ripen bananas, store them in a brown paper bag with an already ripe fruit. Keep in a cool, dark place.

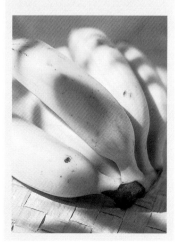

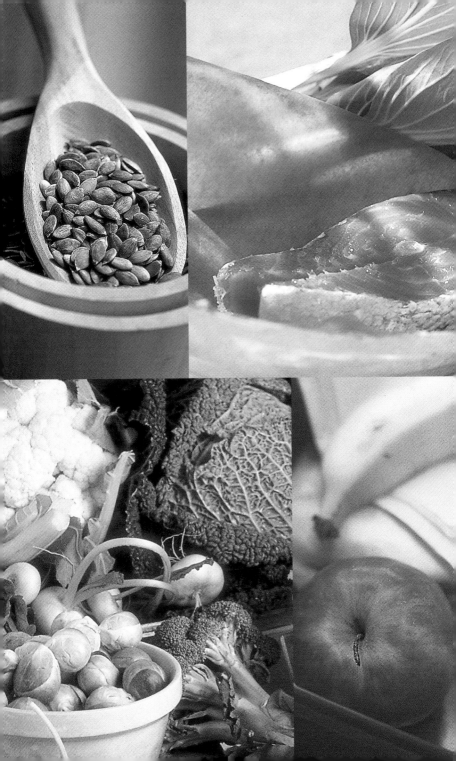

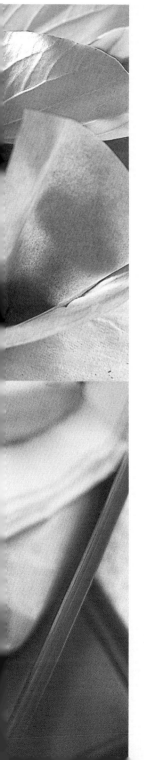

# foods that heal

Eating a well-balanced diet, with plenty of fruit and vegetables, gives you the best possible basis for good health. Even so, there will be times when you will succumb to coughs and colds, wake up with a headache, or feel a bit down in the dumps.

The good news is that eating specific foods can be of enormous help in easing all sorts of everyday ailments, either by helping the immune system to work more efficiently, supplying essential nutrients that have been lacking in the diet, or by helping to restore balance to a body system that is under stress.

A little of what you fancy may do you good!

# easing the symptoms

**If you are not in peak physical condition, the signs often show in the body. Dull, lifeless locks don't necessarily mean merely a bad hair day; they may signal that something more serious is wrong.**

Thin or brittle nails, successive mouth ulcers, digestive upsets   all these are indications that all is not as it should be. The problem may be something minor, a health hiccup if you like, but it is also possible that there is a more serious underlying cause. Always see your doctor if symptoms persist or are particularly severe. This book offers some suggestions that may help to prevent certain conditions from developing, and ease those that have, but it is not our intention to suggest that diet can ever be a substitute for professional diagnosis and treatment.

Having said that, there are plenty of practical steps you can take to ease unpleasant symptoms. Imagine sipping a glass of papaya juice next time you have a sore throat. As it goes down, the cool

▼ ALTERNATIVE HEALTH PRACTITIONERS CAN HELP YOU COME TO TERMS WITH AN ILLNESS OR CONDITION BY SUGGESTING DIETARY AND LIFESTYLE CHANGES THAT WILL HELP.

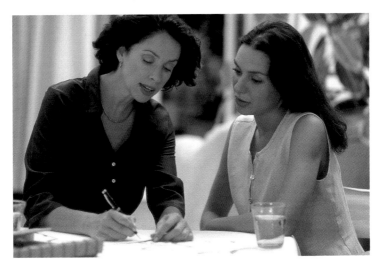

liquid will soothe and comfort, and an enzyme in the fruit will help to alleviate your discomfort. If you have had a bout of diarrhoea, eating live yogurt can help to balance the microflora in the gut. A ripened banana can boost potassium levels and help to bring down high blood pressure.

Nature provides a wonderful natural pharmacy of fruits, vegetables, herbs and spices, which can be of great benefit alongside conventional medical treatment.

▾ EXERCISING HELPS TO KEEP YOU FIT, REDUCES STRESS AND TENSION AND MAKES YOU FEEL BETTER PSYCHOLOGICALLY.

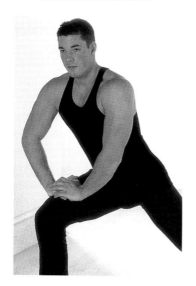

## RECIPE SUGGESTION

PAPAYA JUICE SOOTHER

This reviving juice helps the throat, liver and kidneys.

*INGREDIENTS*

*1 papaya*

*½ cantaloupe melon*

*90g/3½oz white grapes*

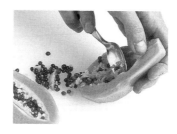

**1** Halve and skin the papaya, remove the seeds and cut into rough slices. Cut open the melon and remove the seeds. Slice the flesh away from the skin, then cut into rough chunks.

**2** Blend the fruit in a processor.

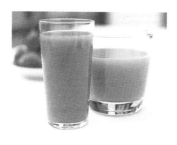

# headaches & migraine

**Having a headache is no fun, and when headaches occur regularly, or are particularly severe, they can be worrying as well as unpleasant. If you notice a recurring pattern to your headaches, you need to take action.**

If your doctor has ruled out any underlying medical condition, making changes to your diet can make you less prone to headaches, particularly if they are triggered by low blood sugar levels. Erratic eating habits can be a factor, so eat small amounts of healthy food at regular intervals, and don't skip meals.

If you wake up with a thumping headache after a night out, you may be dehydrated so drink plenty of water. Coffee and cola contain caffeine, which affects the blood supply to the brain, and can cause headaches, so drink in moderation.

Tension headaches – the kind that make you feel as though your head is trapped in a vice – may be caused by stress. Make sure you are getting your quota of B vitamins by eating wholegrains, dairy products, lean meat, seafood, green vegetables, nuts and seeds. Vitamin C is depleted in times of stress, so eat an orange or a couple of kiwi fruit every day.

## MIGRAINE

Some migraine attacks appear to be triggered by a reaction to a specific food, with chocolate, cheese, coffee and citrus fruits the main culprits. Alcohol, especially red wine, may also be implicated, and there are some suggestions that stock cubes, processed meats that contain nitrates and even pulses (legumes) can be problematical for some sufferers. Food allergies can be a trigger; if you think this may be the case, seek advice.

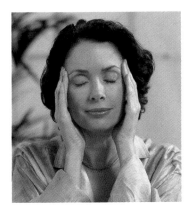

◄ DON'T IGNORE A HEADACHE, PARTICULARLY IF YOU ARE A REGULAR SUFFERER.

# colds & sore throats

**Colds are especially common in winter, and characterized by streaming eyes, a sore throat, blocked nose, headaches, aching muscles and a high temperature. Getting plenty of rest and taking care of your health will speed your recovery.**

A healthy lifestyle, plenty of exercise and a balanced diet won't stop you getting coughs and colds, but it will help to build up your resistance. You are also likely to recover more rapidly than someone who is below par. If you do succumb, the best advice is to drink plenty of fluids, alternating water with fresh citrus juices. There is some evidence that foods that are rich in zinc can help you fight off a cold. Oysters are the best source, but may not slide down a sore throat all that readily. Try soft scrambled eggs, another source of zinc.

A hot toddy with lemon is an old favoured recipe based on sound nutritional sense. Lemons, like limes, are rich in vitamin C, and have potent antiseptic qualities, making them ideal for combating sore throats and sniffles. Alternatively, try papaya juice, which is great for soothing a sore throat. Reduce dairy produce, which tends to increase mucus production.

If your throat is fine, and you just have a heavy cold, a curry may be just what you need. Include ginger, which is an expectorant, and chilli, a powerful decongestant.

▾ REGARDED AS ONE OF LIFE'S LUXURIES, OYSTERS ARE RICH IN ZINC.

▾ EGGS PROVIDE B VITAMINS, VITAMINS A AND D, AND IRON.

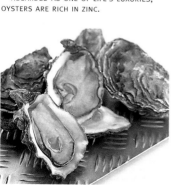

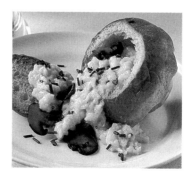

# a healthy digestive system

**To break down food we need friendly bacteria and diges-
tive enzymes. These are produced by the stomach and small
intestine and can get out of balance due to poor diet, stress,
antibiotics, food intolerances or toxin overload.**

If we suffer these conditions then
food remains semi-digested and
conditions such as constipation,
nausea, flatulence and indigestion
can arise. If you are prone to
digestive problems, avoid spicy
foods, alcohol and processed
foods, which can all irritate the gut.

## CONSTIPATION

This is a common problem. If there
is no underlying medical condition,
it may be the result of poor diet,
inadequate fluid intake and a

▼ GINGER CAN HELP TO SOOTHE STOMACH
CRAMPS. TRY A GINGER AND PEPPERMINT TEA.

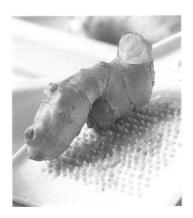

sedentary lifestyle. If you make sure
you get enough fibre, drink plenty
of water and take some exercise,
symptoms can often be alleviated
naturally, which is better than
resorting to laxatives.

Fresh fruit and vegetables,
which are good sources of soluble
fibre, stimulate the digestive
system, but avoid beans, cabbage
and Brussels sprouts, which can
cause flatulence and indigestion.
Other foods that can boost your
fibre levels are brown rice, dried
fruit, wholegrain bread and pasta.
Bananas are also useful. They are
a natural, gentle laxative, and can
help to prevent and treat indigestion, and also ulcers.

Eating live natural yogurt can
improve the condition of the gut
and treat gastro-intestinal disorders. Live yogurt contains active,
beneficial bacteria, which balance
the intestinal microflora and
promote good digestion, boost the
immune system and increase
resistance to infection.

# irritable bowel syndrome (ibs)

**It is important to see a doctor if you think you may be suffering from IBS, as similar symptoms may indicate other medical conditions. Symptoms include stomach cramps, bloating, constipation and diarrhoea.**

If you have been diagnosed with IBS, there are several steps you can take, such as eating live yogurt, which may make you more comfortable. Have plenty of fruit and vegetables, which contain soluble fibre, but avoid cabbage, lentils and beans. Avoid insoluble fibre, such as wheat bran, particularly in break-fast cereals. Also make sure you drink six glasses of water every day.

Linseed can be helpful. Dissolve 15ml/1 tbsp linseeds in 250ml/8fl oz/1 cup warm water and leave overnight. Next morning, strain into a mug and drink the liquid.

In some people, IBS may be linked to food intolerance. If you suspect this, seek professional advice. An elimination diet may help to pinpoint the problem – a nutritionist should advise you.

### TIP
To treat a digestive upset, try grated apple or a glass of apple juice.

▼ HERBAL TEAS, ESPECIALLY CHAMOMILE OR PEPPERMINT, CAN HELP IBS.

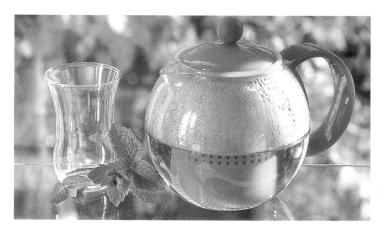

# healthy hair & scalp

**Glossy, shiny hair is synonymous with good health, a fact that manufacturers of shampoo capitalize upon. The first step to beautiful hair and a healthy scalp is to eat a well-balanced diet, with plenty of fresh fruit and vegetables.**

Aim for a good balance of protein foods, including dairy produce, nuts and pulses (legumes). Your shopping list should include organic artichokes, sweet potatoes, carrots, spinach, broccoli, asparagus and beetroot (beet). Choose apricots, citrus fruits, kiwi fruit, berries and apples. Have plenty of oily fish, and shellfish. Drink six glasses of water a day, and limit sugar.

Dry hair and an itching, flaky scalp may be the result of zinc deficiency. The most efficient way to address this is to swallow an oyster (a single oyster yields 18mg zinc, more than most people consume in a day). Other forms of shellfish are good sources of zinc, too, as are red meat and pumpkin seeds. Essential fatty acids in vegetable oils, nuts and oily fish can also improve the condition of the scalp, while the minerals in sea vegetables, such as kombu and arame, help to make hair lustrous.

Vitamins A and B are important if hair is to be shiny and healthy. Eating liver once a week is a great way of boosting your intake of vitamin A (retinol), provided that you are not pregnant. Fish liver oils are the richest source of retinol, but it can be obtained from eggs and full-cream milk. Also eat carrots, spinach, sweet (bell) peppers, sweet potatoes, peaches and dried apricots on a regular basis. These contain betacarotene, which the body converts to vitamin A.

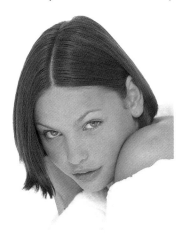

◀ GLOSSY HAIR IS ONE OUTWARD SIGN OF A HEALTHY PERSON.

# improving your skin

**The skin is the largest organ of the body, and is especially vulnerable to the effects of modern living. The most useful thing you can do to improve the quality of your skin is to drink water; ideally six to eight large glasses every day.**

Also of benefit is regular exercise and plenty of fresh air, so a bracing walk in the country is ideal. If you have a specific skin condition, such as eczema or acne, it is important to consult your doctor, but if you merely think your skin is looking a bit lifeless and could do with a lift, you may find the following advice helpful.

Eat fresh vegetables, especially carrots, spinach, broccoli and sweet potatoes, which deliver the antioxidant betacarotene. Citrus fruit, kiwi fruit, berries (especially strawberries), avocados, vegetable oils, wholegrains, nuts, seeds and some types of seafood provide the antioxidant vitamins C and E, selenium and zinc, which help to transport nutrients to the skin and maintain collagen and elastin levels. Zinc-rich foods, such as liver, pate and eggs, can improve conditions such as psoriasis and eczema.

Apples are rich in pectin, which helps to cleanse the liver, thus aiding detoxification of the skin.

Artichokes are good liver cleansers, too, along with asparagus and raw beetroot (beet). Fish, meat and eggs provide B vitamins, which promote a glowing complexion and combat dryness. Similar benefits are to be gained from eating oily fish such as mackerel, salmon, tuna, sardines and herrings. The fatty acids these fish contain (also found in nuts, seeds and vegetable oils) soften and hydrate the skin.

▼ A GLASS OF WATER WITH A SLICE OF LEMON KICK-STARTS THE LIVER.

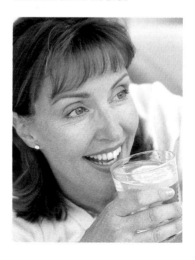

# mouth ulcers

**Having a mouth ulcer may not be a major life problem, but it can make you feel pretty miserable as you worry it with your tongue, or try to avoid chewing close to the affected area and biting it with your teeth.**

What causes these agonizing little spots is not always clear. They can be the result of an iron deficiency, or failure to take in enough B vitamins, but they might be linked to pre-exam nerves or a similar stressful event. Ill-fitting dentures may be to blame, or a broken tooth. They can also be triggered by a food intolerance.

If you suffer from recurrent clusters of mouth ulcers, it is a good idea to see your doctor, as they may be symptoms of disease.

Take a look at your diet, too. It may be helpful to increase your intake of B vitamins by eating more wholegrains, pulses (legumes), meat and milk. Liver is particularly useful, and will also boost your iron intake, especially if eaten with a source of vitamin C. Liver also contains folate, which is essential for the formation of new body cells, and helps to keep the lining of the mouth healthy. Other sources are pulses, wholegrain cereals and green vegetables.

▼ WHOLEGRAIN CEREALS ARE KNOWN TO HELP PREVENT MOUTH ULCERS.

▼ YOU MAY BE MORE SUSCEPTIBLE TO MOUTH ULCERS IF YOU ARE FEELING LOW.

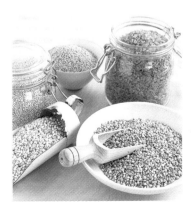

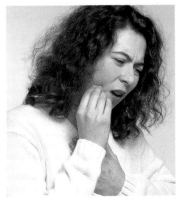

# healthier nails

**Our nails reveal quite a lot about our state of health. Ideally, they should be strong, well shaped and flexible. The nail bed should be pale pink, indicating that the blood is adequately oxygenated.**

The best way to ensure nails are strong and healthy is to eat a balanced diet, with plenty of fresh fruit and vegetables.

◀ SEAWEED AND SHELL-FISH CONTAIN ZINC.

so a meal of braised liver with onions and cherry tomatoes once a week may work wonders. Chickpeas and tofu are a good choice for vegetarians. It used to be thought that drinking milk – or eating cheese – was good for nails, because of the calcium these foods deliver, but this is inaccurate. Nails are made of a protein called keratin and contain little calcium.

Drink lots of water, and make sure that you get enough iron, which helps to prevent the nails fromthinning. Foods that are good sources of iron include liver and other red meat, fish, poultry, green leafy vegetables, dried apricots, prunes and wholegrain cereals. To optimize iron absorption, eat suitable foods with ingredients that deliver vitamin C, such as tomatoes or potatoes, or drink orange juice with your meal. Avoid drinking tea, as the tannin impairs iron absorption.

If your nails are dry and brittle, you may not be getting enough zinc. Seafood (especially oysters), eggs and liver are good sources,

Wide ridges on the nails can indicate a deficiency of selenium, which is closely associated with the function of vitamin E in the body. Good sources are meat, especially liver, fish and shellfish, chicken and wholegrain cereals. Don't worry if you find little white spots on your nails – these are not sinister, and probably indicate minor damage, such as knocking against a table.

# anxiety & stress

**It is almost impossible to avoid stress. A hectic workplace, unrealistic demands on our time, trying to juggle a job and care for a family, facing a life change such as retirement – all these elements make it increasingly difficult to cope.**

If you are severely stressed, it is all too easy to bottle it up. Counselling can be beneficial or you may need medication. There are also some simple ways you can help yourself. A nutrient-rich diet combined with regular exercise and a healthy lifestyle can help to reduce anxiety levels. Your diet should include wholegrains, dairy products, liver, green vegetables, seafood, lean meat, nuts, seeds, yeast extract, pulses (legumes), eggs and forti-fied breakfast cereals. These are all good sources of B vitamins, which help the body cope with stressful situations, and correct poor sleep patterns. Vitamin C is depleted in times of stress, so eat citrus fruit, kiwi fruit, broccoli, potatoes and green leafy vegetables. Magnesium levels may be low, too: wholegrain cereals, nuts, pulses, sesame seeds, sea vegetables, dried figs and leafy green vegetables can help to restore the balance. Eating oily fish can also be beneficial, especially if you include the bones. This deliv-ers a double benefit: omega-3 fatty acids and calcium for efficient func-tioning of the nerves.

Being stressed can affect health in many different ways. The most immediate, and obvious, is its effect on digestion. Taking time over meals, making sure you are relaxed when eating, eating a balanced diet with plenty of fruit and vegetables, and drinking lots of water can only help.

▲ SARDINES ARE A HEALTHY OILY FISH.

# minor depression

**It is no coincidence that we crave sweet foods when we are feeling down. Studies show that sweet, carbohydrate foods, like biscuits, chocolate and cakes, help in the production of seratonin, a neurotransmitter that is said to lift the spirits.**

Bingeing on sugary foods affects blood sugar levels, and a quick high will soon be followed by a deep low. The answer is to eat complex carbohydrates, like wholemeal (whole-wheat) bread, muffins or scones, cereal bars, brown rice or wholemeal pasta, which are broken down slowly in the body. They will give you a seratonin lift, but its effects will be even and last longer.

The amino acid tryptophan, which the body converts to seratonin, is found in lean meat, poultry, eggs, soya beans and some other pulses (legumes), dried dates, broccoli, low-fat dairy products, bananas and watercress, so next time you are feeling just a bit blue, chop up a banana with a couple of dried dates and eat it with a spoonful of low-fat yogurt. Sprinkle over a few Brazil nuts and you add selenium, a mood enhancer.

Not getting enough iron can lead to mild depression, so make sure you are getting enough of this valuable mineral, remembering that vitamin C is needed if the body is to absorb it properly.

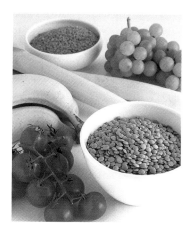

◀ FRUIT, PULSES (LEGUMES) AND VEGETABLES HELP TO KEEP BLOOD SUGAR LEVELS STABLE.

## QUICK LIFT
Chillies stimulate the brain to release endorphins, which naturally boost the spirits. Ginger has a similar effect, so a meal of stir-fried chicken, liver or tofu with fresh root ginger and chillies is a savoury solution to feast upon if you are feeling down.

# diabetes

**The incidence of diabetes in the Western world is increasing. Many cases of the milder form of this disease are not diagnosed, or are diagnosed too late to prevent some lasting damage, so it is important to be aware of the symptoms.**

Diabetes is the result of the body's inability to control the amount of glucose in the blood. An essential form of energy, glucose is produced when we digest starchy and sugary foods. Blood glucose levels rise until a certain level is reached, whereupon the pancreas releases insulin to bring the levels back to normal. If the pancreas fails to produce insulin, Type 1 – insulin-dependant diabetes – is the result. If the body fails to utilize insulin correctly, or the pancreas becomes inefficient, Type 2 – sometimes referred to as adult-onset diabetes – occurs. Symptoms of untreated diabetes include thirst, frequent urination, headaches, blurred vision, weight-loss or nausea.

All diabetics need to control their diet with professional help. To keep blood sugar levels under control, it is vital to eat a balanced, healthy diet, and to lose any excess weight under medical supervision. The diet should be high in high-fibre, starchy carbohydrates, which raise blood glucose levels gradually and maintain them for longer. Wholemeal (whole-wheat) bread, potatoes, rice and pasta are recommended. It is important to eat five portions of vegetables and fruit daily, but very sweet fruit should only be eaten occasionally, because of the fructose they contain. Diabetics who are not overweight may be able to eat very small amounts of sugar in food, but

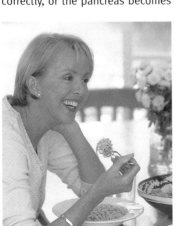

◀ EATING SMALL REGULAR MEALS WILL HELP KEEP YOUR BLOOD SUGAR LEVELS STEADY.

should avoid sweets and sweetened drinks. A low-fat diet is essential, as diabetics have an increased risk of coronary heart disease. Salt should be limited.

It is important to eat regular meals. Grazing – eating little and often – may be a good approach for Type 2 diabetics, helping to keep blood sugar levels steady.

## QUICK BEAN FEAST RECIPE SUGGESTIONS

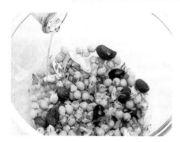

• Mix cooked chickpeas with spring onions (scallions), olives and chopped parsley, then drizzle over a little olive oil and some lemon juice.

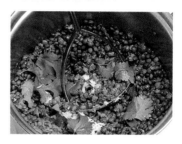

• Mash cooked beans with olive oil, garlic and coriander (cilantro) and pile on to toasted wholemeal (whole-wheat) bread. Top with a poached egg.

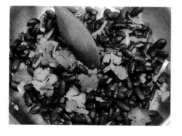

• Heat a little olive oil and stir-fry cooked red kidney beans with chopped onion, chilli, garlic and fresh coriander leaves.

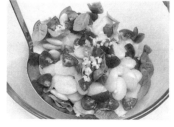

• Dress cooked beans with extra virgin olive oil, lemon juice, crushed garlic, diced tomato and fresh basil.

# restless legs

**This may sound like a puppet's problem. The syndrome usually occurs when you sit or lie down. The legs jerk involuntarily and there may be discomfort, "pins and needles" or a burning pain.**

The problem is often at its worst at night, making it difficult for sufferers to get to sleep. The cause is unknown, but there is some evidence that RLS (restless leg syndrome) can be inherited. It can also begin at any age. Women who suffer from it may find their symptoms worsen when they are pregnant or in later years during the menopause.

It may help to choose a diet that is rich in iron. Liver, dried apricots, prunes and wholegrain cereals are good sources (avoid liver if you are pregnant). Folate, which is essential for building new body cells, can also ease the symptoms, so eat liver, pulses (legumes), green vegetables and wholegrain cereals. It is also worth increasing your intake of vitamin B12 by eating lean meat and dairy produce.

RLS may worsen as you age. It can be linked to circulatory problems, so the diet should include foods that are rich in vitamin E, such as avocados and beansprouts.

## RECIPE SUGGESTION

SPICED APRICOT PURÉE
Try this with natural yogurt.

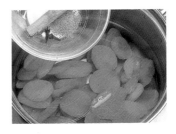

**1** Place 350g/12oz/1½ cups dried apricots in a pan with water to cover. Add 1 cinnamon stick, 2 cloves and 2.5ml/½ tsp freshly grated nutmeg. Simmer until soft.

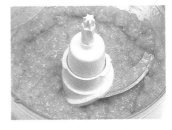

**2** Remove the cinnamon stick and cloves. Leave to cool, then purée until smooth.

# fatigue

**Are you often exhausted, too weary even to contemplate getting undressed for bed? Do you fall asleep on your desk after lunch? Have you been known to wake up feeling weary or as if you need a good night's sleep?**

All the above are typical of chronic fatigue, which can be linked to a medical condition such as diabetes, and must be investigated by a doctor. General tiredness, however, is something all of us suffer from time to time. It may be unavoidable, the result of sleepless nights getting up to a small baby, or studying hard for an exam, or it may be linked to depression or a similar emotional state.

There may be a physical explanation, such as iron deficiency.

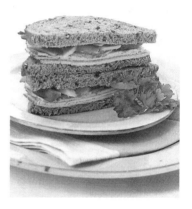

▲ COMPLEX CARBOHYDRATES PROVIDE AND SUSTAIN CONSTANT ENERGY LEVELS. CHOOSE BREADS CONTAINING WHOLEGRAINS.

## ENERGIZE

If your energy levels have taken a dive because your blood sugar is low, don't reach for a bar of chocolate or a rich biscuit. The quick energy boost these give will be followed by a slump, and you may end up far more tired than you were at the start. Eat a wholemeal (whole-wheat) salad sandwich instead; the carbohydrate in the bread will give you a more efficient energy fix that will be more prolonged and even.

This can happen when a woman has particularly heavy periods. To redress the balance, eat iron-rich foods such as dried apricots, liver, red meat, pulses (legumes), eggs, green leafy vegetables, fortified breakfast cereals, seeds and wholegrains. At the same time, eat citrus fruit, kiwi fruit or blackcurrants. These are good sources of vitamin C, which is necessary for the uptake of iron into the bloodstream.

# joint problems

**Aching joints are a common problem, especially as we get older. The condition may be related to a recognized medical condition, such as rheumatoid arthritis or osteoarthritis, but may simply be down to general wear and tear.**

Whatever the cause, aching joints are no fun. Simply straightening up or getting in and out of a car can be very uncomfortable. There is a lot of discussion as to whether diet has any role to play in the prevention or treatment of either condition, but several recent studies suggest that antioxidants and oily fish may help.

▼ DOING TOO MUCH GARDENING, OR TAKING UNACCUSTOMED EXERCISE CAN MAKE YOUR JOINTS STIFF AND UNCOMFORTABLE.

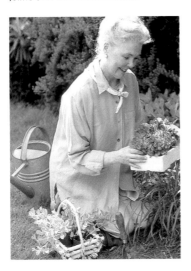

ARTHRITIS

The most common forms of this condition are rheumatoid arthritis and osteoarthritis. The former is a complex condition whose cause is largely unknown. It is an inflammatory condition affecting the joints and is thought to be related to a malfunctioning immune system. It can strike at any age. Osteoarthritis is a degenerative condition of the joints, which most commonly occurs with age, and tends to affect those who are overweight. Certain foods may bring relief to arthritis sufferers, but others can make the symptoms worse. If this happens, an allergy may be implicated. Consult an expert, who may recommend you try an exclusion diet, followed by a tailor-made diet plan.

You can boost your antioxidant intake by eating plenty of green leafy vegetables, also carrots, broccoli, sweet potatoes and avocados, which contain appreciable amounts of vitamins C and E, betacarotene and selenium. Apricots, apples,

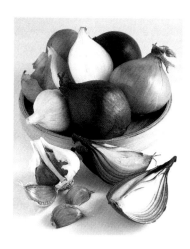

▲ Onions are one of the oldest natural cures. They stimulate the body's antioxidant mechanisms and help arthritis, rheumatism and gout.

sufferers and may help those with osteoarthritis. It is certainly worth eating oily fish more often (about three times a week is recommended) as there are other health benefits too. The vitamin B12 in oily fish is important for a healthy nervous system, and the iodine promotes healthy thyroid function. Fish oils are rich in omega-3 fatty acids, which can help to reduce inflammation. Vegetarians should eat soya beans, tofu, linseeds, wheatgerm, walnuts and rapeseed oil: all good alternative sources of omega-3 fatty acids.

It has been suggested that New Zealand green-lipped mussels may help to reduce inflammation, although there is limited therapeutic evidence of this.

bananas and mangoes are the best fruits to eat. Try eating asparagus and celery, both of which have anti-inflammatory properties, and may help to reduce swelling and ease painful joints. Another anti-inflammatory agent is quercetin, which is found in kelp, onions and apples. Spices that have anti-inflammatory qualities include turmeric and fresh root ginger.

## Eat More Oily Fish
Salmon, tuna, mackerel, sardines and herrings have been shown to offer relief to rheumatoid arthritis

▼ Cook fish the healthy way — try grilling (broiling), poaching or baking it.

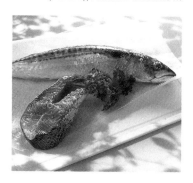

# women's health

**Fluctuating hormone levels have a marked effect on women's wellbeing. Balance can be easier to achieve if you adopt a healthy lifestyle, enjoy plenty of regular exercise and watch what you eat.**

PRE-MENSTRUAL SYNDROME (PMS)
Any woman who regularly experiences pre-menstrual syndrome (PMS) will need no explanation of the symptoms. Mood swings, irritability, food cravings, bloating, constipation and diarrhoea can all occur, and when these symptoms are every month, 2–14 days before a period starts, life can be difficult.

Certain foods may offer some benefits. Wheatgerm, wholegrains, bananas, oily fish and poultry are

▾ TAKING PLENTY OF EXERCISE AND EATING A BALANCED DIET WILL HELP RELIEVE PMS.

good sources of vitamin B6, which is especially helpful in combating water retention and breast tenderness. Vitamin B6 can aid the absorption of magnesium, a lack of which causes mood swings and cravings. Magnesium is found in fruits and vegetables. Jacket potatoes (with the skin) are an excellent source, as are avocados and Chinese leaves (Chinese cabbage). Dried apricots, liver, red meat, eggs, green leafy vegetables, seeds and wholegrains are rich in iron, a lack of which can lead to anaemia and

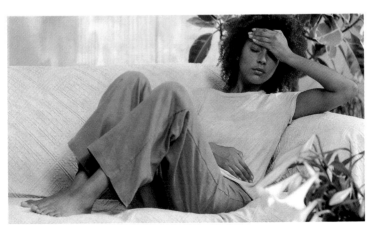

fatigue. To help the body absorb iron, take in plenty of vitamin C, such as kiwi fruit and blackcurrants.

Breast pain can cause discomfort. It may be eased by eating foods rich in essential fatty acids such as oily fish, sunflower oil, rapeseed oil, nuts and seeds, or by eating foods rich in vitamin E such as vegetable oils, nuts, avocados, eggs and wheatgerm.

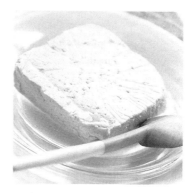

▲ TOFU IS AVAILABLE IN DIFFERENT FORMS, AND CAN BE USED IN SOUPS, SALADS AND STIR-FRIES.

## MENOPAUSE

Some women sail through the menopause, but others experience side effects, such as depression, insomnia and anxiety, hot flushes, vaginal dryness and night sweats. These symptoms can be eased by HRT (hormone replacement therapy), but a healthy diet may help.

There is current interest in the role of phytoestrogens – chemicals in plants that act in a similar way to the female hormone, oestrogen. Japanese women, whose diets are high in phytoestrogens, have few menopausal problems and a lower risk of breast cancer. It is hoped that trials will confirm whether eating more phytoestrogen-rich food – soya beans, tofu, soy milk and linseeds – can help Western women.

It is believed that soya products may help to maintain bone density and also reduce the risk of breast cancer. Sweet potatoes contain natural progesterone, and may help to correct hormone imbalance and ease menopausal symptoms. To slow down bone density loss during menopause, eat calcium-rich foods like low-fat dairy products, nuts, seeds, green leafy vegetables, canned fish, pulses, seaweed and bread. Foods rich in vitamin D, zinc and magnesium are also valuable.

Treat yourself to an avocado now and then. This vegetable is rich in potassium, which helps to prevent fluid retention, and is high in vitamin E, which may help to alleviate hot flushes.

# a healthy heart

**What you eat has a direct bearing on the health and efficiency of your heart and circulatory system. You may not be able to do anything about hereditary heart disease or stroke, but you can eat sensibly, take exercise and avoid obesity.**

Reducing the amount of saturated fat you consume is a vital first step. Limit dairy products, fatty meat and hydrogenated or trans fats found in margarine and processed foods. Foods high in saturated fats are chocolates, cakes, sauces, biscuits (cookies) and puddings. Saturated fat may be listed as hydrogenated vegetable fat or oil.

Eat plenty of fresh fruit and vegetables. The fibre, phytochemicals, antioxidants and vitamins they

▼ EATING FOODS HIGH IN VITAMIN E CAN HELP TO IMPROVE THE CIRCULATORY SYSTEM.

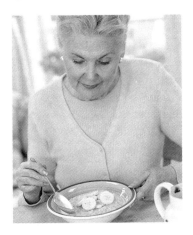

contribute help to prevent the furring-up of the arteries. Green, leafy vegetables and pulses (legumes) are high in folate, which reduces levels of homocysteine. This amino acid has been linked to increased risk of coronary heart disease and strokes. Eat one or two garlic cloves a day. Garlic has been found to lower blood cholesterol levels, reduce blood pressure and help to prevent blood clots forming.

Omega-3 oils have the same effect. You'll find these in oily fish, walnuts, wheatgerm and soya beans. Just one serving of oily fish a week is believed to cut the risk of heart attack by half.

Eat oats, lentils, nuts and pulses. The insoluble fibre they contain can reduce blood cholesterol levels when eaten as part of a low-fat diet.

Red wine, tea and onions all contain the flavonoid quercetin, which may reduce the risk of heart disease and strokes. Drink wine in moderation only.

# boosting the immune system

**A healthy immune system is the key to maintaining general good health and keeping infections at bay. Poor diet and stress have a negative effect on the immune system, leaving the body vulnerable to colds, flu and disease.**

A diet based on unprocessed foods, along with a healthy lifestyle, is essential for maintaining the immune system. Raw fruits and vegetables, especially sprouting seeds, are particularly helpful.

Key protective foods include good sources of the antioxidant vitamins C and E, and betacarotene, which help to boost the immune system. Sweet potatoes and avocados are ideal, as are berry fruit (especially blackcurrants) and citrus fruit. Limes and lemons are also good for colds, coughs and sore throats, and have potent antiseptic properties.

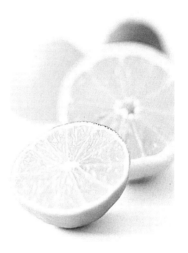

▲ CITRUS FRUITS ARE A RICH SOURCE OF VITAMIN C.

## PUMPKIN SEEDS

Boost your zinc intake with pumpkin seeds by
• Sprinkling them over baked goods before cooking.
• Adding them to flapjacks.
• Tossing them into a stir-fry.
• Adding them to a sweet crumble topping.
• Using them to make pesto.
• Scattering them over a salad.

Also good are wholegrains, meat, tuna, salmon, nuts, seeds and bananas, which provide vitamin B. This supports the body's production of antibodies. Zinc is an essential mineral to boost and support a healthy immune system. It can be found in shellfish such as oysters and crab, eggs, beef, turkey, pumpkin seeds, peanuts, cheese and yogurt.

# food allergy & intolerance

**Food does not always heal. Food sensitivities – allergies and intolerances – seem to be on the increase, and can cause anything from minor discomfort to serious risk in susceptible individuals.**

An allergic reaction is not the same as a food intolerance. The former occurs when the body reacts to an essentially harmless substance as though it were an invading organism like a bacterium. An immune response is triggered and antibodies are activated to deal with the threat. What happens next depends on the individual, the site of the problem and the allergen itself.

Sneezing and watering eyes are common, as are hives, asthma and eczema. Sometimes the reaction is violent, and can be life threatening, as is the case with peanut allergy.

Food intolerance is more subtle, occurring when the body finds a substance difficult to cope with. Why this should happen is not always clear, but when the offending food is located and omitted

▼ TRY TO ELIMINATE ONE FOOD AT A TIME FROM YOUR DIET AND NOTE ANY CHANGES.

▼ AN ORANGE JUICE ALLERGY DOESN'T MEAN YOU CAN'T EAT OTHER CITRUS FRUITS.

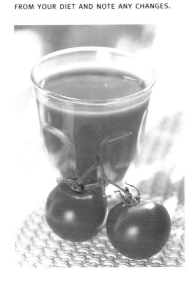

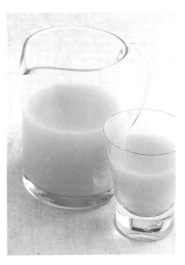

from the diet, the results can be quite dramatic.

There are many different types of food intolerance. Among the common culprits are soya products, caffeine, chocolate, orange juice, tomatoes and food additives. The lactose in cow's milk and the gluten in wheat, rye and barley are often implicated. The symptoms are wide ranging, but can include anxiety, depression, fatigue, headaches, skin disorders, asthma, joint or muscle pain, rheumatoid arthritis and mouth or stomach ulcers. Irritable bowel syndrome can be linked to a food intolerance.

It is one thing to suspect a food allergy or intolerance; quite another to track it down. Seek advice from a doctor, dietician or naturopath.

## ALTERNATIVES

If you are lactose intolerant, try switching to soya milk, but make sure you get sufficient calcium from other sources. Live yogurt can often be tolerated, as the bacteria in the yogurt helps to break down the lactose.

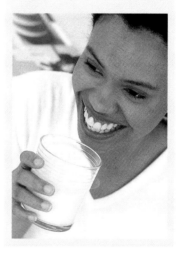

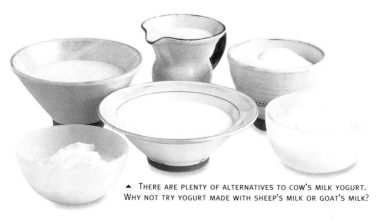

▲ THERE ARE PLENTY OF ALTERNATIVES TO COW'S MILK YOGURT. WHY NOT TRY YOGURT MADE WITH SHEEP'S MILK OR GOAT'S MILK?

# glossary

**Amino acids** These are the basic components of proteins. There are 20 in all, 12 of which can be synthesized by the body and eight which must come from our food.

Quinoa, pronounced "keen-wa", is the only known complete food, in that it contains all eight of the essential amino acids that the body cannot make. Usually our bodies obtain them from a variety of foods.

**Antioxidants** Found in vitamins A, C and E, in co-enzyme Q10 and betacarotene, as well as in minerals like selenium and zinc, these help to mop up free radicals in the body, thus limiting tissue damage.

**Betacarotene** is what gives fruit and vegetables such as mangoes, apricots, carrots, (bell) peppers and sweet potatoes their bright orange colour. An important antioxidant, betacarotene can be converted into vitamin A by the body.

**Carcinogens** are cancer-causing substances.

**Complex carbohydrates** These are contained in fresh fruit, wholemeal (whole-wheat) bread, fruit bread, wholemeal muffins or scones, wholegrain cereal, brown rice and wholemeal or buckwheat pasta. The body breaks complex carbohydrates down slowly, providing sustained energy over a long period of time. Complex carbohydrates can also promote sleep if they are eaten towards the end of the day.

**Enzymes** These are protein molecules that act as catalysts in the body, making it possible for biological processes to take place. Metabolic enzymes are implicated in the building of healthy bones, tissues and muscle. Digestive enzymes, most of which come from the food we eat, ensure that food is digested and made available to the body, or eliminated. Enzymes are

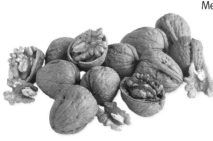

vital for every biological function and poor enzyme activity can seriously damage our health.

**Essential fatty acids** Fatty acids are responsible for several bodily processes, including the maintenance of cell walls. The body can manufacture most fatty acids, but two main types – essential fatty acids – must come from food. These are omega-3, found in oily fish, walnuts and rapeseed oil; and omega-6, from corn oil and sunflower oil. These fats are "good" fats, and should be eaten regularly. In effect they help the body to process damaging fats.

**Free radicals** These are damaging molecules produced by the body as part of a natural process. The chemical structure of a free radical differs from a healthy molecule in that it has an unpaired electron. The electron roams the body searching for a healthy electron to pair up with. This process damages

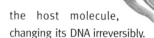

the host molecule, changing its DNA irreversibly. Free radicals only survive for a short time, but if they exist in large numbers they can cause extensive cell damage resulting in heart disease, cataracts and cancer. Eating foods rich in antioxidants eliminates free radicals from the body.

**Goitre** is a painful swelling of the thyroid gland.

**Phytochemicals** are plant compounds, widely found in fruit and vegetables, which appear to offer protection against diseases like cancer, arthritis, heart disease and hypertension, and may slow down the ageing process. Phytochemicals also have antioxidant properties.

**Phytoestrogens** These are chemicals found in plants. They mimic the action of the female sex hormone, oestrogen, and can be helpful in reducing menopausal symptoms. Soya beans are a good source.

# essential vitamins & minerals

| VITAMIN | BEST SOURCES | ROLE IN HEALTH |
|---|---|---|
| **A** (retinol in animal foods, beta-carotene in plant foods) | Milk, butter, cheese, egg yolks and margarine, carrots, apricots, squash, red (bell) peppers, broccoli, green leafy vegetables, mango and sweet potatoes. | Essential for vision, bone growth and skin and tissue repair. Beta-carotene acts as an antioxidant and protects the immune system. |
| **B1** (thiamin) | Wholegrain cereals, brewer's yeast, potatoes, nuts, pulses (legumes) and milk. | Essential for energy production, the nervous system, muscles and heart. Promotes growth and boosts mental ability. |
| **B2** (riboflavin) | Cheese, eggs, milk, yogurt, fortified breakfast cereals, yeast extract, almonds and pumpkin seeds. | Essential for energy production and for the functioning of vitamin B6 and niacin as well as tissue repair. |
| **Niacin** (part of B complex) | Pulses, potatoes, fortified breakfast cereals, wheatgerm, peanuts, milk, cheese, eggs, peas, mushrooms, green leafy vegetables, figs and prunes. | Essential for healthy digestive system, skin and circulation. It is also needed for the release of energy. |
| **B6** (piridoxine) | Eggs, wholemeal (whole-wheat) bread, breakfast cereals, nuts, bananas and cruciferous vegetables, such as broccoli and cabbage. | Essential for assimilating protein and fat, to make red blood cells, and a healthy immune system. |
| **B12** (cyanocobalamin) | Milk, eggs, fortified breakfast cereals, cheese and yeast extract. | Essential for formation of red blood cells, maintaining a healthy nervous system and increasing energy levels. |
| **Folate** (folic acid) | Green leafy vegetables, fortified breakfast cereals, bread, nuts, pulses, bananas and yeast extract. | Essential for cell division. Extra is needed pre-conception and during pregnancy to protect foetus against neural tube defects. |
| **C** (ascorbic acid) | Citrus fruits, melons, strawberries, tomatoes, broccoli, potatoes, peppers and green vegetables. | Essential for the absorption of iron, healthy skin, teeth and bones. An antioxidant that strengthens bones. |
| **D** (calciferol) | Sunlight, margarine, vegetable oils, eggs, cereals and butter. | Essential for bone and teeth formation, helps the body to absorb calcium and phosphorus. |
| **E** (tocopherol) | Seeds, nuts, vegetable oils, eggs, wholemeal bread, green leafy vegetables, oats and cereals. | Essential for healthy skin, circulation and maintaining cells – an antioxidant. |

| MINERAL | BEST SOURCES | ROLE IN HEALTH |
| --- | --- | --- |
| Calcium | Milk, cheese, yogurt, green leafy vegetables, sesame seeds, broccoli, dried figs, pulses, almonds, spinach and watercress. | Essential for building and maintaining bones and teeth, muscle function and the nervous system. |
| Iron | Egg yolks, fortified breakfast cereals, green leafy vegetables, dried apricots, prunes, pulses, wholegrains and tofu. | Essential for healthy blood and muscles. |
| Zinc | Peanuts, wholegrains sunflower and pumpkin seeds, pulses, milk, hard cheese and yogurt. | Essential for a healthy immune system, tissue formation, normal growth and wound healing and reproduction. |
| Sodium | Most salt we eat comes from processed foods such as crisps, cheese and canned foods. It is also found naturally in most foods. | Essential for nerve and muscle function and the regulation of body fluid. |
| Potassium | Bananas, milk, pulses, nuts, seeds, wholegrains, potatoes, fruits and vegetables. | Essential for water balance, normal blood pressure and nerve transmission. |
| Magnesium | Nuts, seeds, wholegrains, pulses, tofu, dried figs and apricots and vegetables. | Essential for healthy muscles, bones and teeth, normal growth and nerves. |
| Phosphorous | Milk, cheese, yogurt, eggs, nuts, seeds, pulses and wholegrains. | Essential for healthy bones and teeth, energy production and the assimilation of nutrients. |
| Selenium | Avocados, lentils, milk, cheese, butter, brazil nuts and seaweed. | Essential for protecting against free radical damage and may protect against cancer. |
| Iodine | Seaweed and iodized salt. | Aids the production of hormones released by the thyroid gland. |
| Chloride | Table salt and foods that contain salt. | Regulates and maintains the balance of fluids in the body. |
| Manganese | Nuts, wholegrains, pulses, tofu and tea. | Essential component of various enzymes that are involved in energy production. |

# index